Parties make me sick

A story for and about
children
who have problems with food

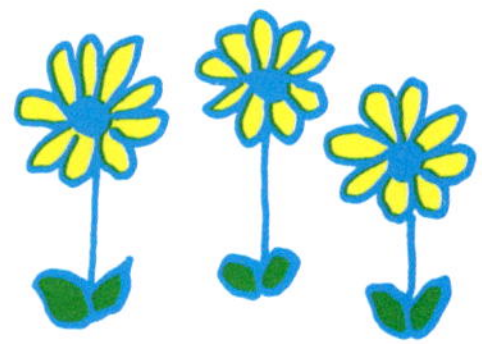

Written by Rae Paterson
Illustrated by Judy McKechnie

About Alma Publications:

Alma Publications is a new venture. We aim to publish low-cost, high quality materials about many aspects of parenting, especially maternal and child health and nutrition. We hope to become a small but locally significant part of the present international network of mother and child health educators, transplanting significant innovations into materials accessible to Australian parents. Our publications will be typeset and printed in Australia—a policy arising not from chauvinism but from an awareness of the human costs of offshore publishing. We invite parent support groups and interested professionals to contact us. Review copies of publications are available free of charge. Our profit margins will be kept as low as possible, and we will offer special reductions to financially disadvantaged groups; hence we will not refuse donations from those able to afford more than the minimum prices set.

Groups ordering 10 or more copies of any of our publications qualify for a handsome discount. Please enquire from Alma Publications, 5 Meredith Crt., Alfredton, 3350.

Published November 1983
National Library of Australia
ISBN 0 9593183 2 1
Printed by The Dominion Press-Hedges & Bell,
Maryborough, Victoria

Preface for Parents

This little book has been written and illustrated by two parents* who,—like you?—know what it means to have a child who is affected by common foods. The medical symptom may be asthma, eczema, diarrhoea, colic, failure to thrive, hives, hyperactivity, learning disability, growing pains, or many other common problems. But once you have identified the food triggering that symptom, the real problem is no longer the symptom. It is the social and very practical problem of persuading your child, your friends and relations, and even teachers and others, that avoidance of some food or foods is in the child's (and family's) best interests. It is also the social handicap of being "different" which seems to be so unacceptable in our conformist society. If this book helps you and your child to see his problem as commonplace and manageable; if it helps provide some understanding of the problem of food intolerance; if it helps some children resist the many temptations offered by ignorant but well meaning adults—it will have been worth the time and effort we all have invested in producing it. We invite your comments.

Maureen Minchin
Author of *'Food for Thought'*

* *Rae Paterson* & *Judy McKechnie* produced the *'Katie'* series, published and distributed by the Nursing Mothers' Association of Australia.

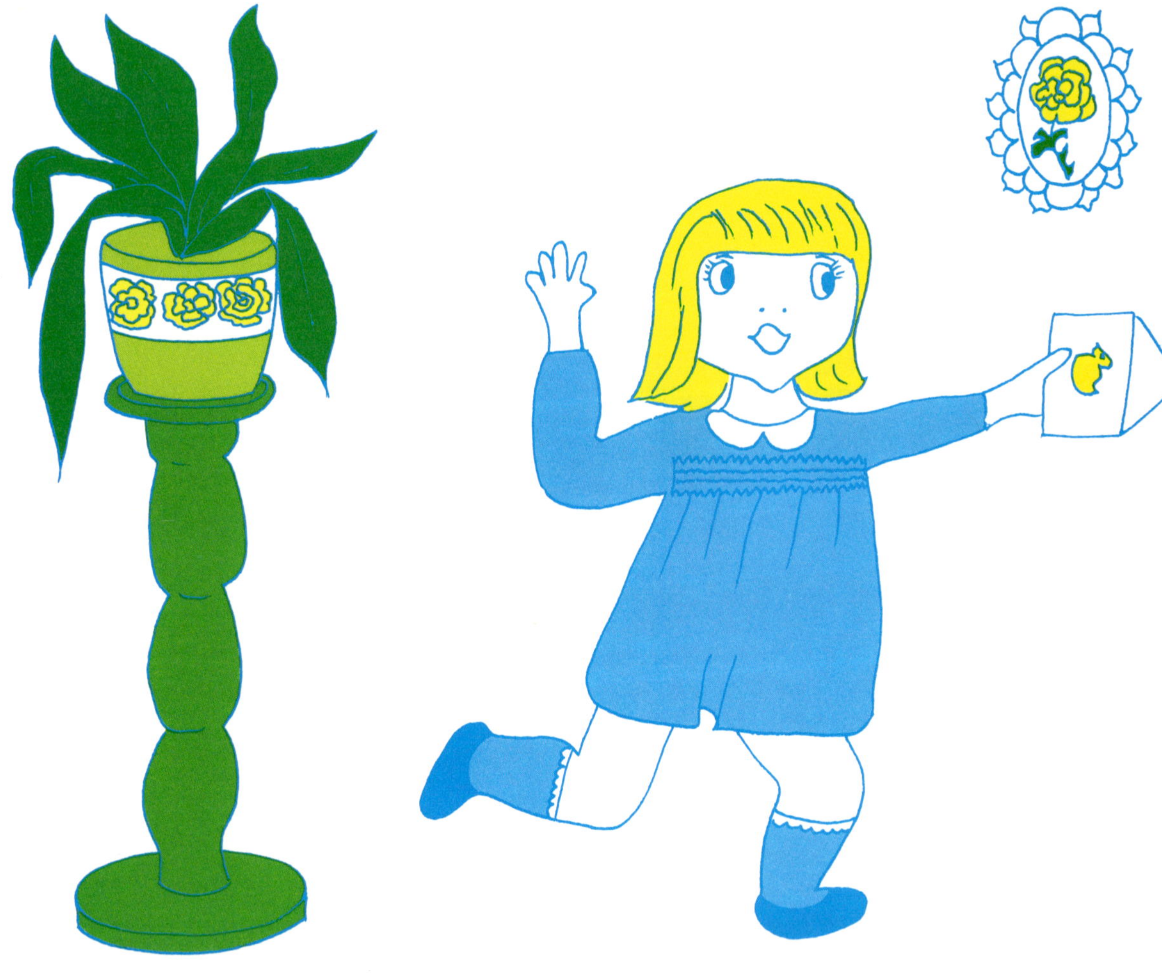

Kirsty was excited. She came rushing in the door and waved an envelope in front of her mother.

"Mum! Michael has invited me to his party. All the kids are going. It will be terrific."

"That sounds interesting," her mother said. She was busy peeling potatoes for tea and wasn't listening too hard.

"Mum, what will I wear? Can I wear my new skirt? I wonder if my blue shoes still fit me?"

Then she stopped.

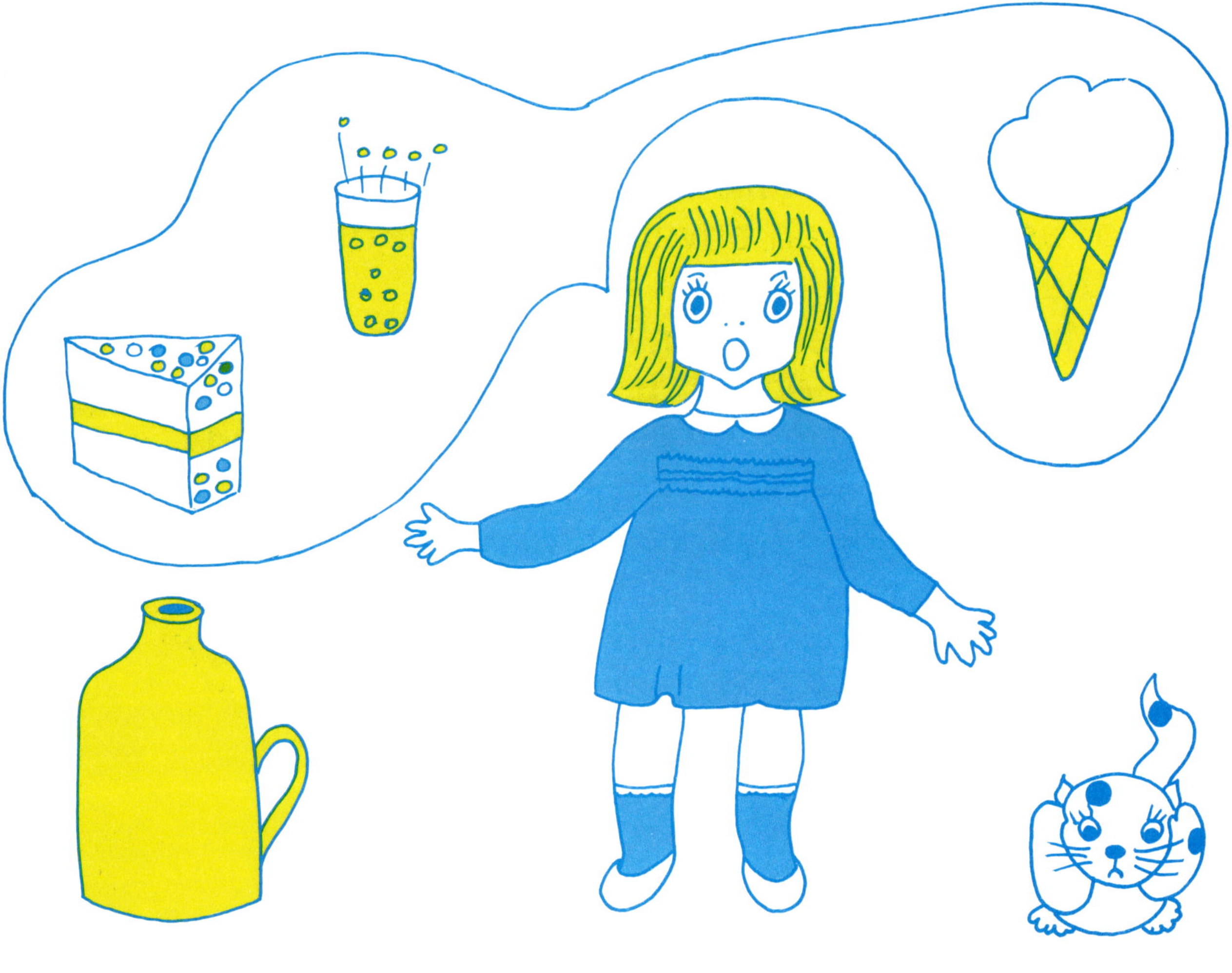

She remembered that she was allergic to lots of party foods. This meant that there were many foods that she couldn't eat because they made her feel sick and uncomfortable.

"Oh mummy!" she cried in despair. "They will have cake, won't they? And I can't eat it. There will be lemonade and ice-cream and I'm not allowed those things. It's not fair!"

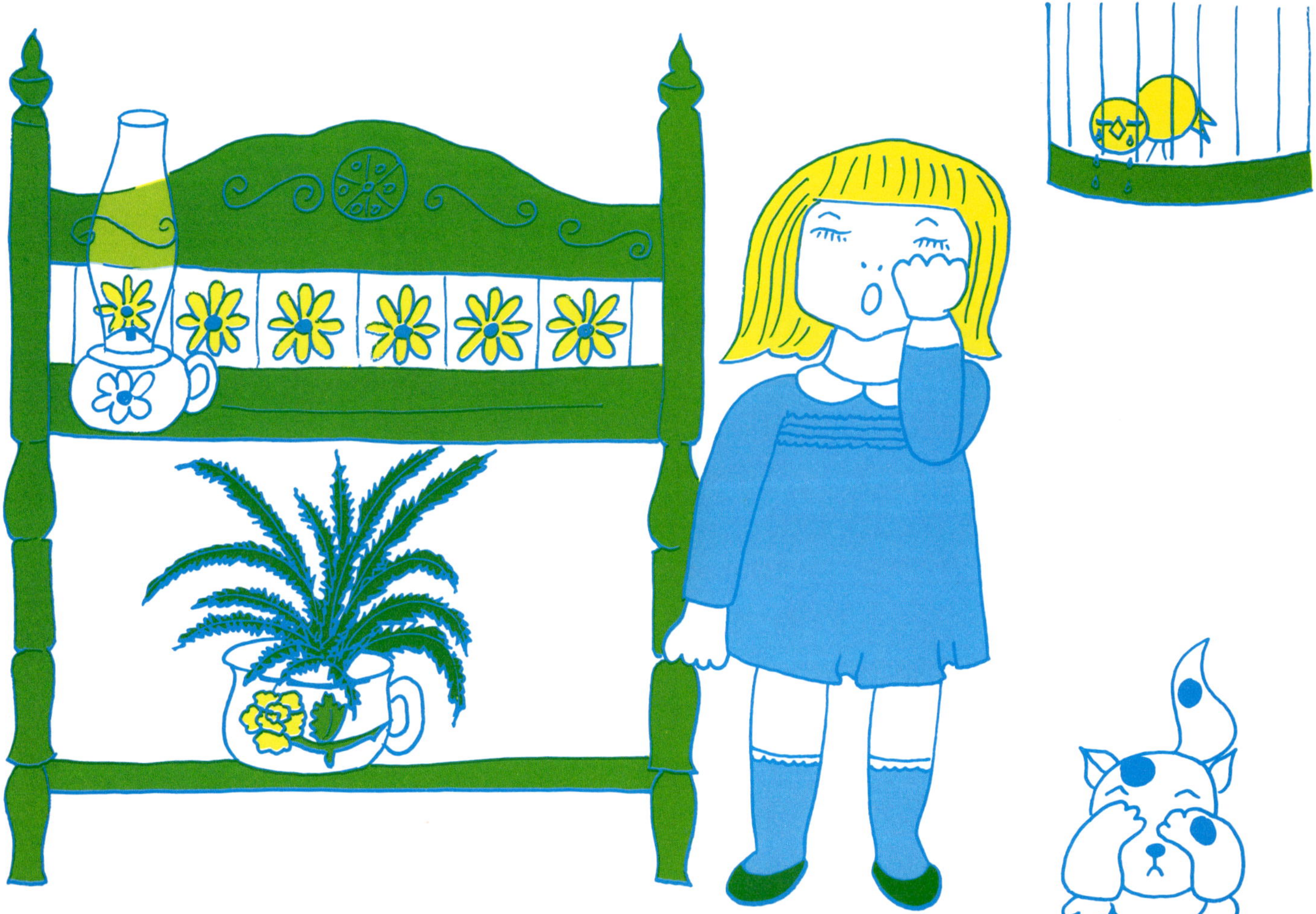

"I know darling," her mother said. "I know how difficult it is for you. I'll make you some special biscuits and you can take your own juice."

"I don't want any special biscuits and nobody else has juice!" Kirsty wailed. "I want to eat the same as everyone else."

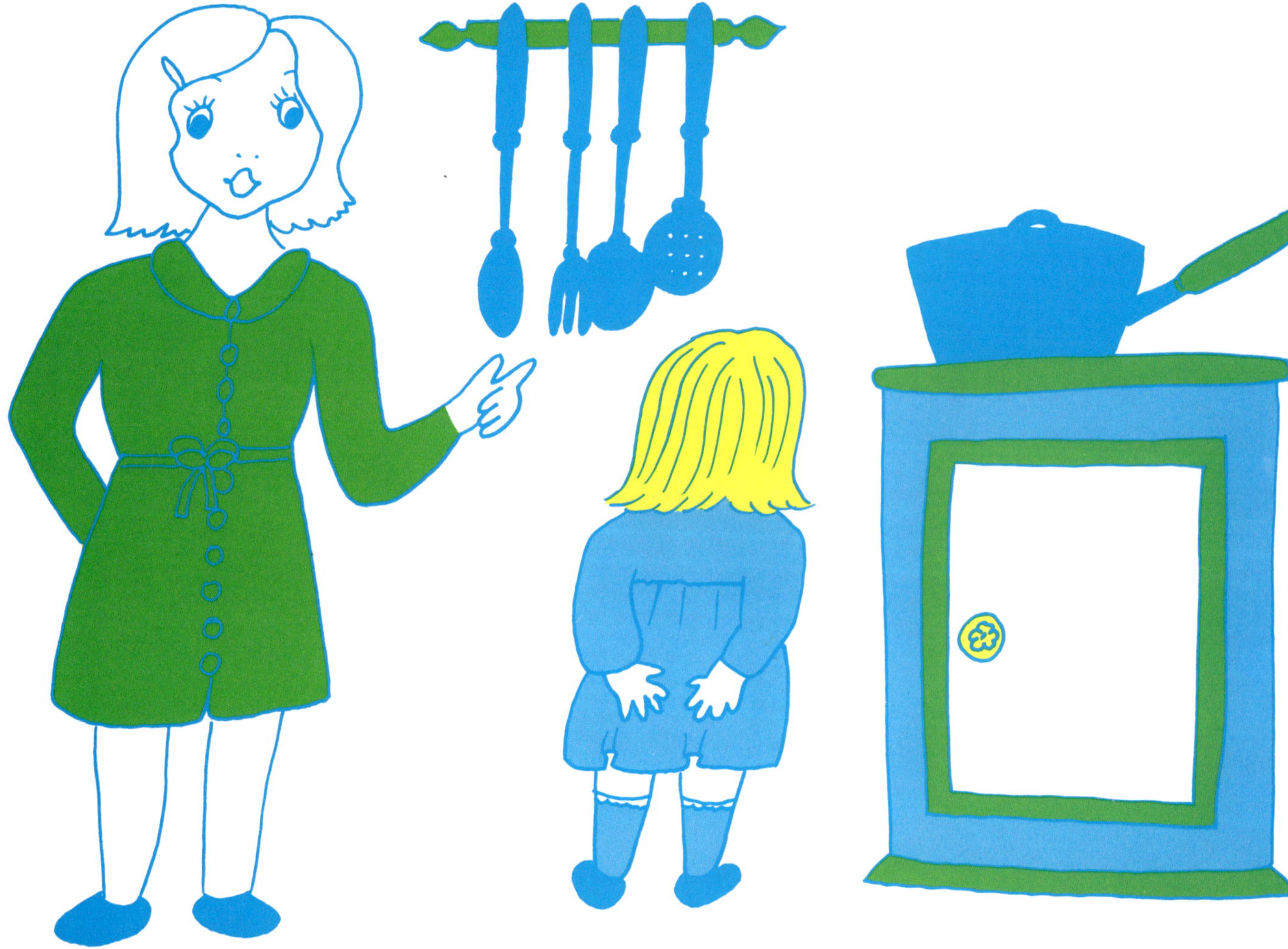

"I know you do, Kirsty," said her mother patiently, "but you know what happens when you eat the wrong food. Remember how awful you feel and how itchy you get?"

"Yes, I know," sighed Kirsty. She remembered very well. How could she forget that terrible itchy rash called eczema, and the tummy pains and headaches she got if she ate the foods she was allergic to?

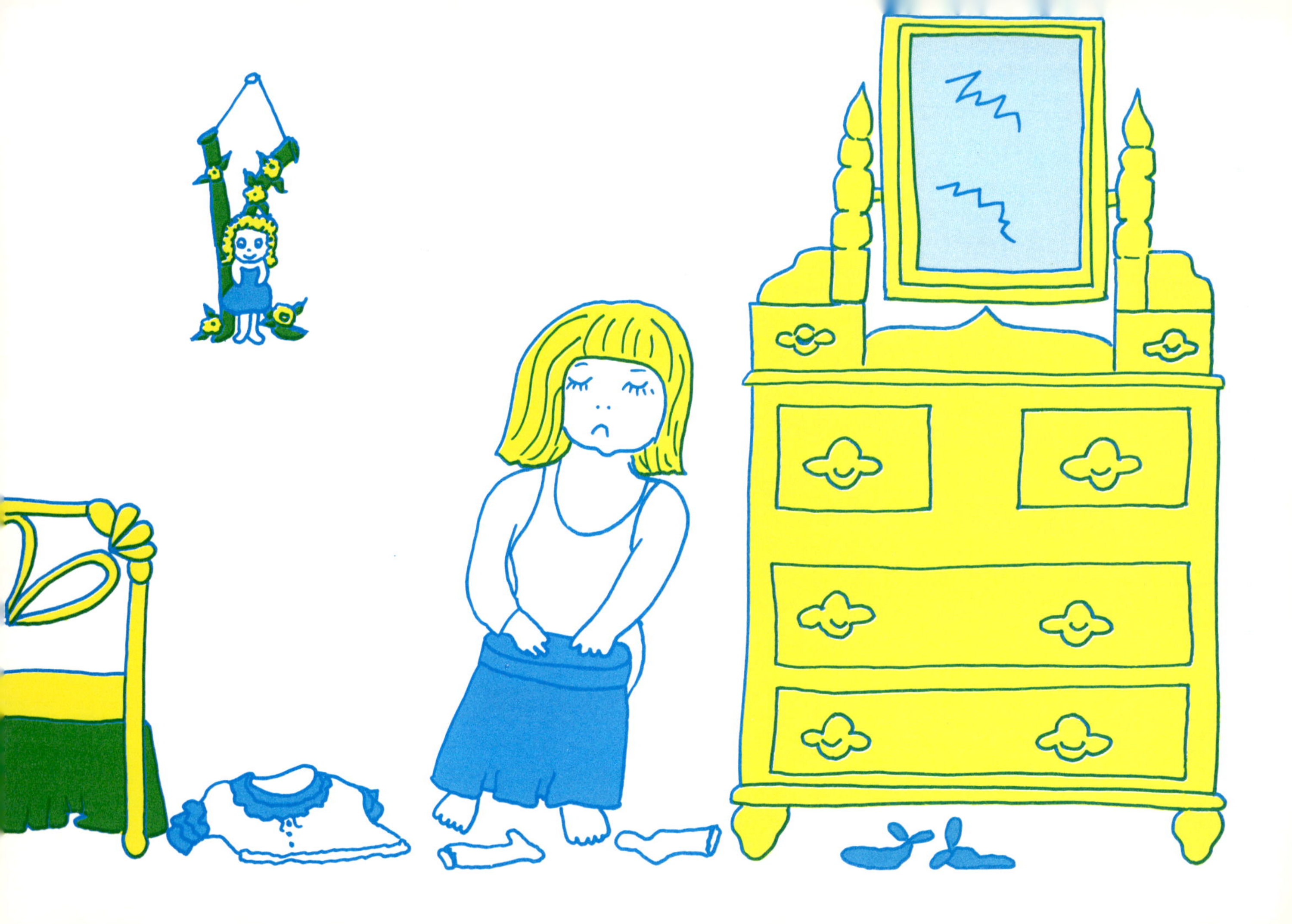

On the day of Michael's party, Kirsty was excited as she put on her new blue skirt. But she was afraid, too. She wondered if Michael's friends would tease her because she couldn't eat the party foods.

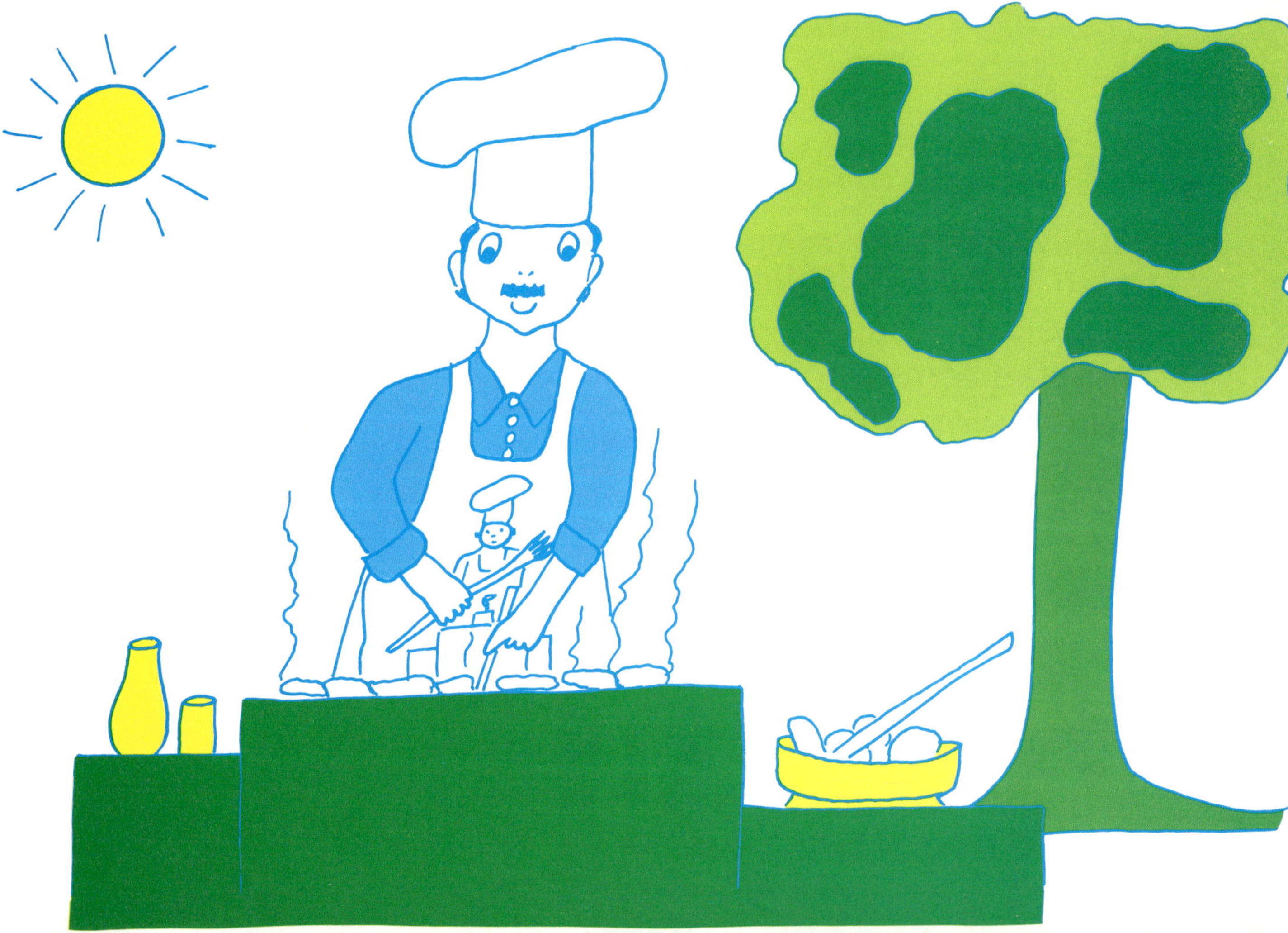

When the mealtime arrived all the children went outside, and there was Michael's dad cooking at the barbecue. Kirsty sighed with relief when she saw the food—meat and salad and apple juice. She was able to eat all those things!

Michael said to her, "I hope you like barbecues. I can't have party food because I'm allergic to sugar and all those flavourings they put in most food. I get asthma," he told her.

Kirsty stared in surprise. Michael was just like her!

"I'm allergic to milk," she told him, "and lots of other foods too. I was frightened I wouldn't be able to eat anything at your party."

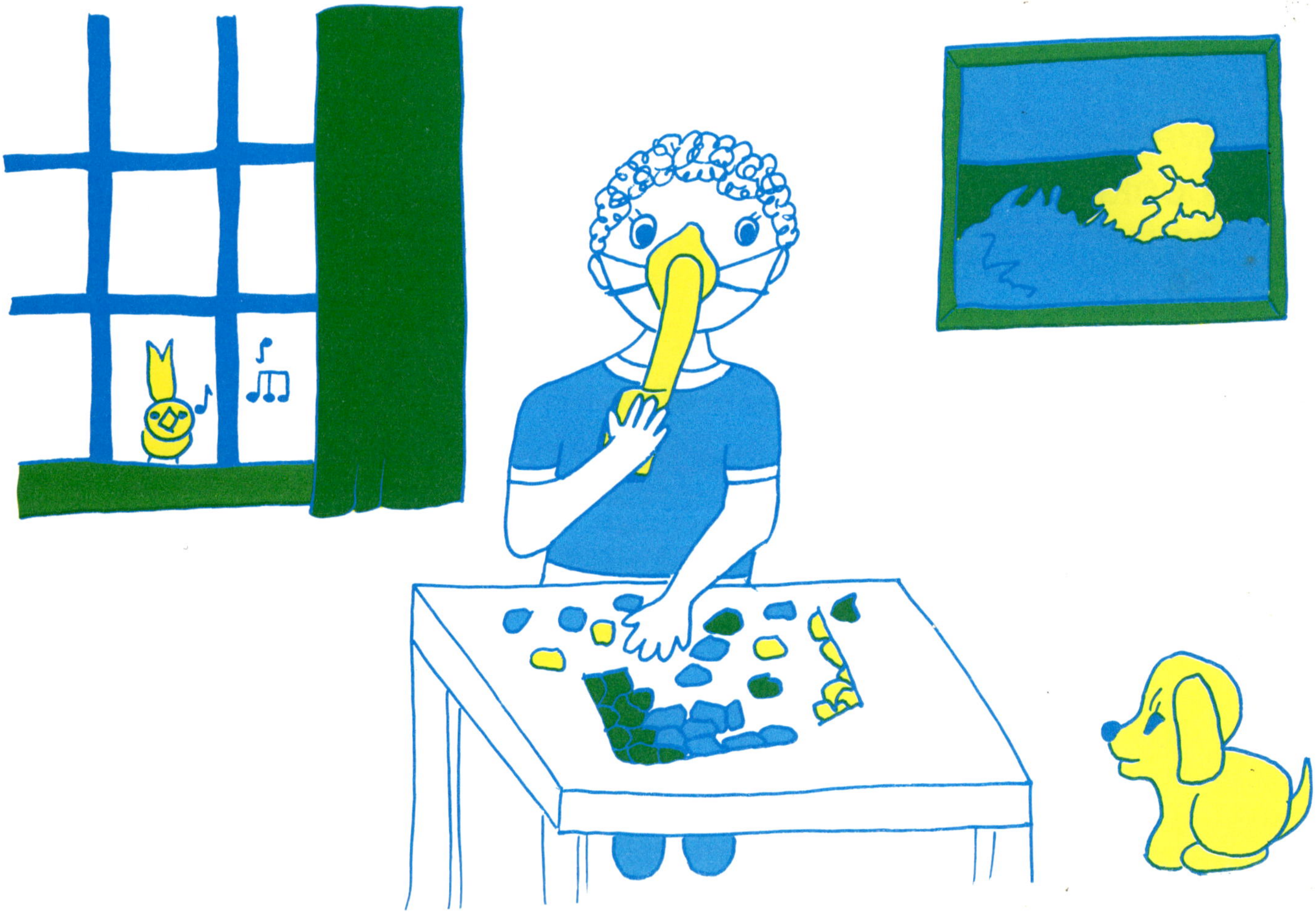

"Michael, what happens when you get asthma?" Kirsty asked.

"I can't breathe properly and I cough a lot," Michael told her. "I have to take special medicine to help me breathe better."

"It sounds frightening," Kirsty decided.

"I don't get it now if I keep on my diet," Michael explained.

"Sometimes I eat things I shouldn't," Kirsty confessed, "then I get eczema again. And sometimes I get a headache and a tummy ache. Then I wish I had kept to my diet."

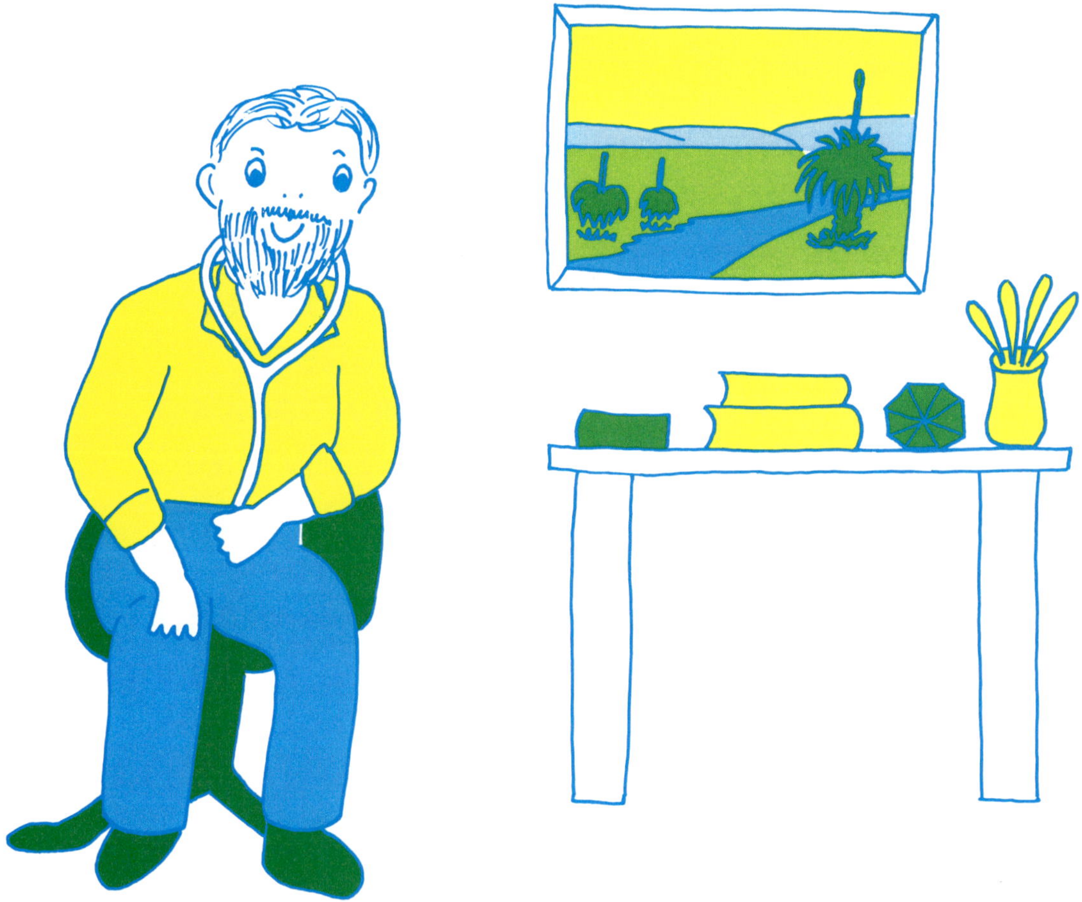

Some of the other children were listening.

"Do you mind being on a special diet?" one of them asked.

"Of course we do!" Michael answered. "But it is better than always being sick."

"I get asthma," said another. "Maybe it's because I'm allergic to something I eat."

"Our doctor says it is really quite common," Kirsty told them. "Lots of kids are allergic to all sorts of things but their parents don't realize it."

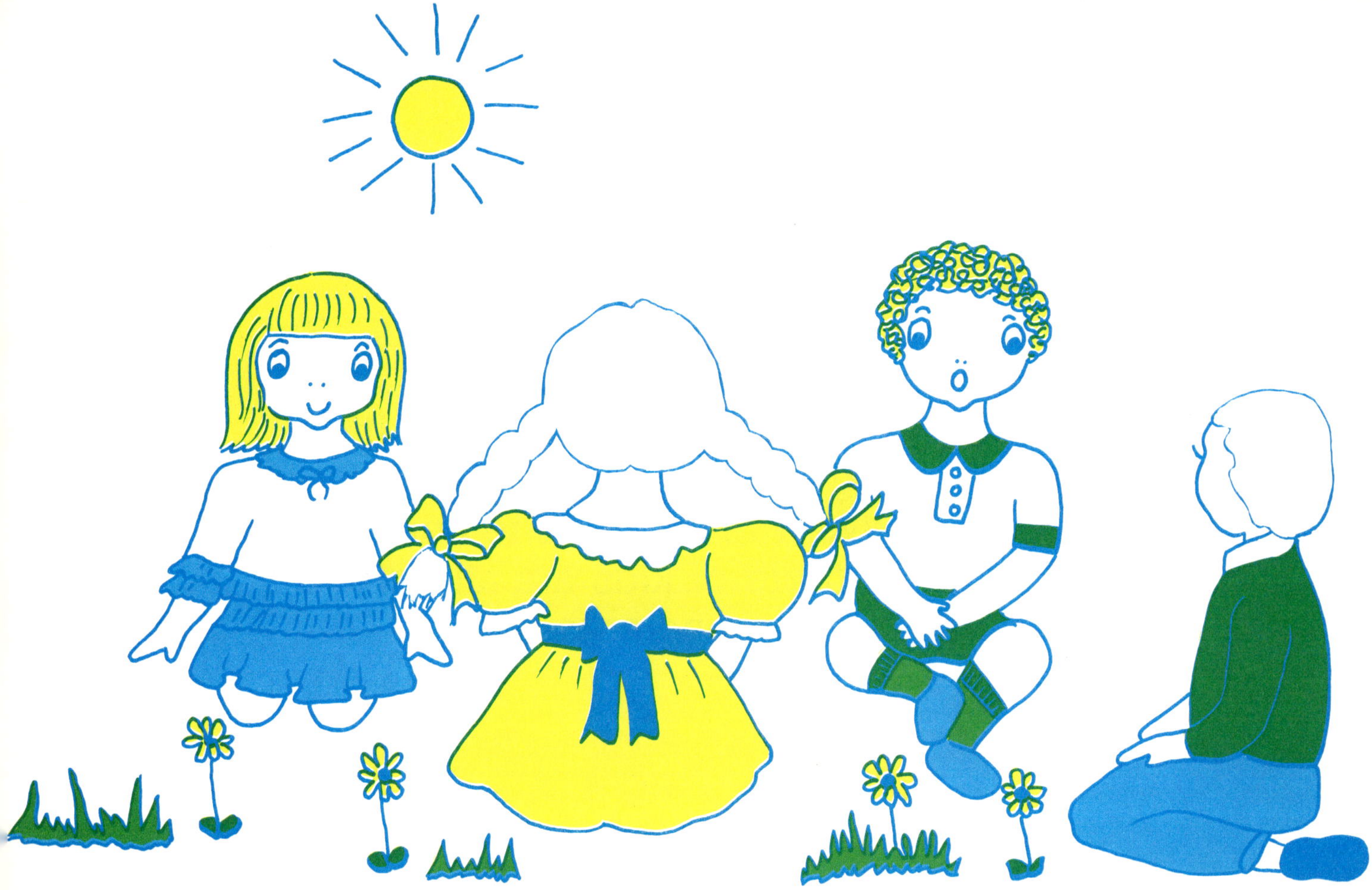

"Do you remember Tony who was always getting into trouble at school last year?" one of the girls asked. "He was hyper-active and could never sit still and do his work. Well, they discovered that he was allergic to foods too, and now that he knows what foods he can't eat, he is much better."

"Yes, that's right!" one of the children agreed. "He is never in trouble now like he used to be. Now I know why!"

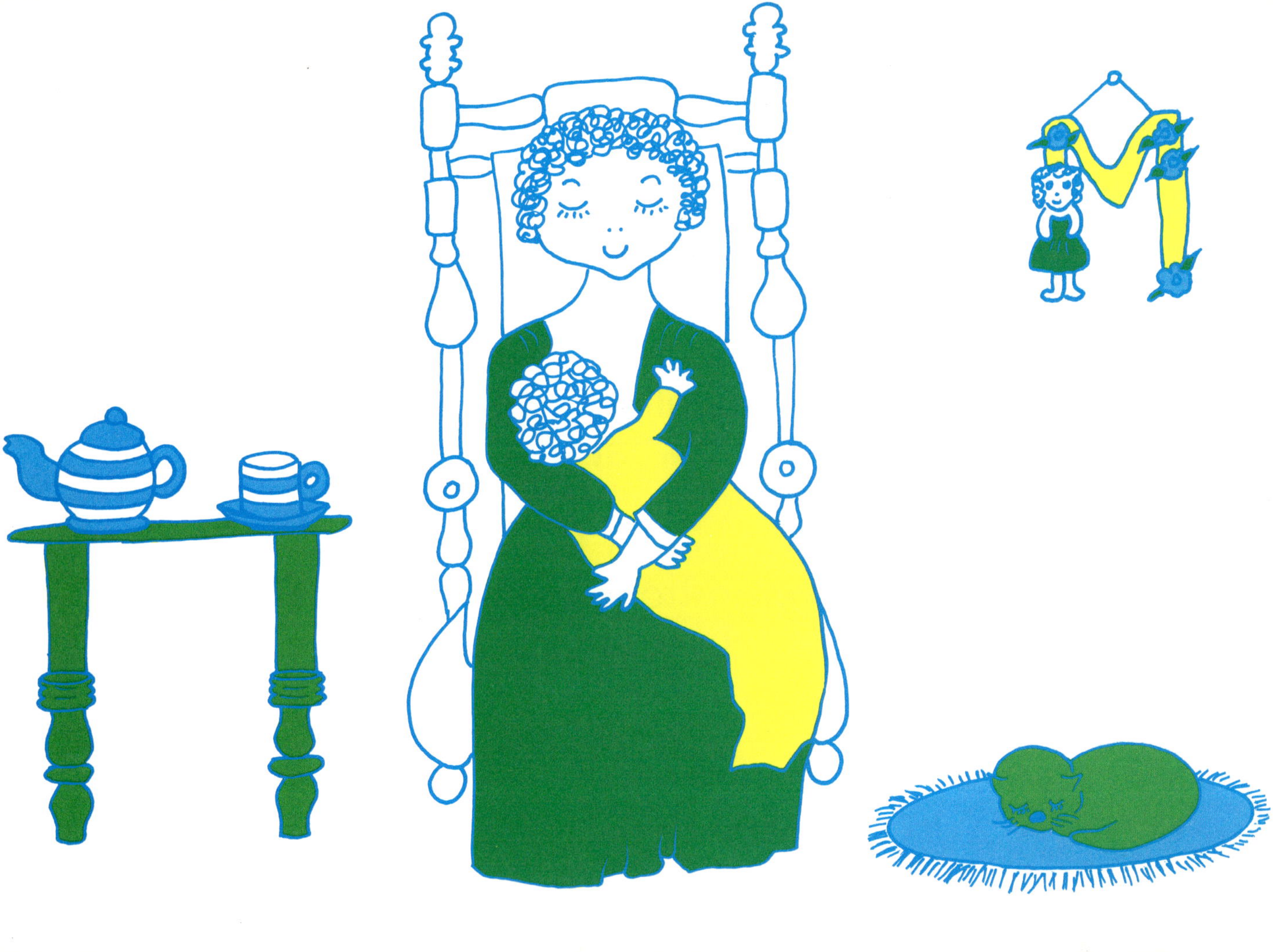

"My dad says that I screamed a lot when I was a baby," Kirsty told them. "People say that all babies cry a lot but I think it is because something is upsetting them, and it might be something they are allergic to."

Michael said, "My mum breastfeeds our baby so that he won't be allergic like me."

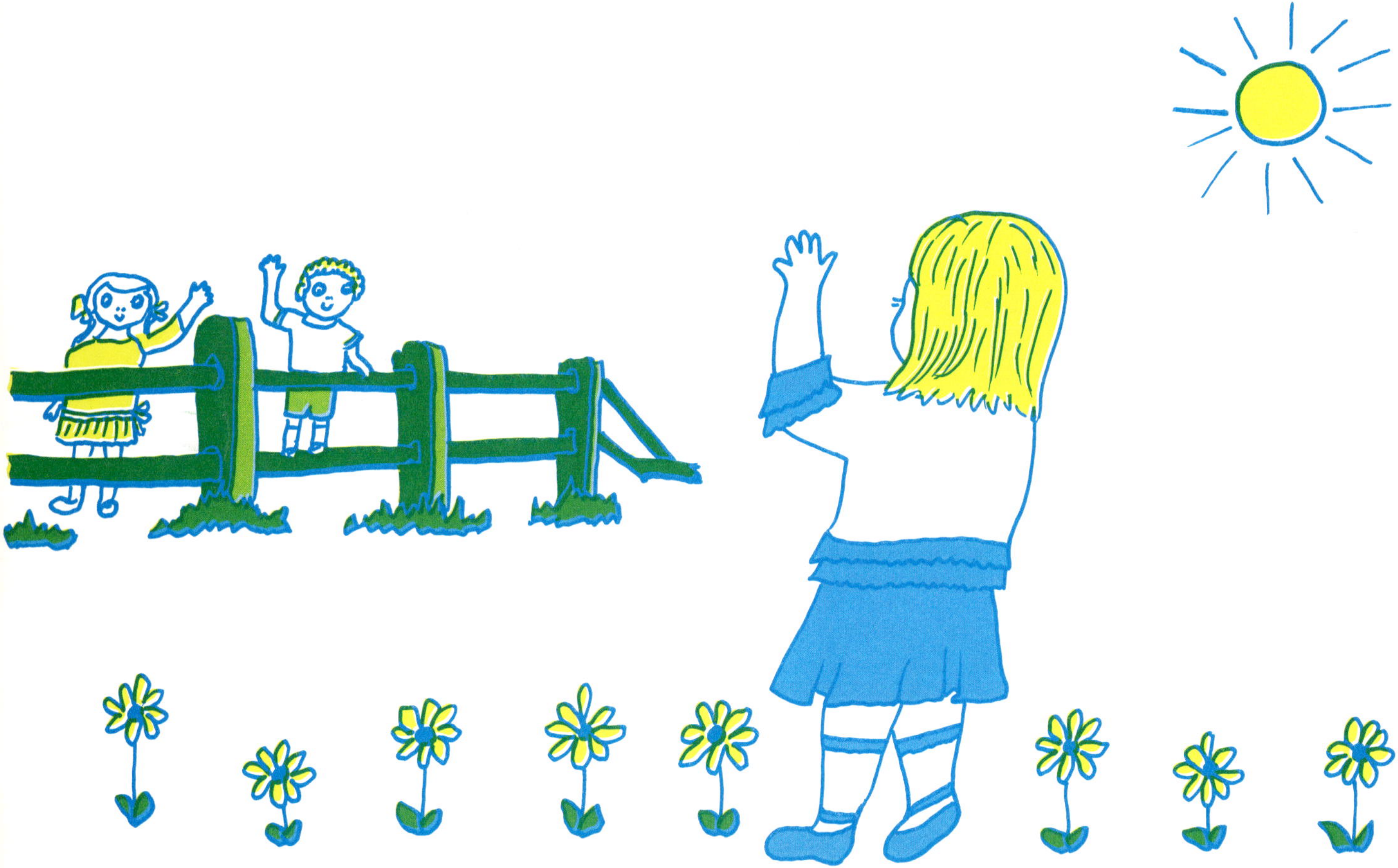

Kirsty was sad when it was time to go home. She was excited to have found someone else who knew what it was like to be on a special diet. She didn't feel so lonely now, and she knew the other children wouldn't ever tease her. They understood her problem.

She decided that parties could be pretty good after all.

Organising a birthday party

A "low-allergy" birthday party is difficult to imagine—birthday parties have come to mean brightly coloured drinks and sweets, ice cream, jelly and lots of cakes. None is necessary and parents with children sensitive to sugar will have long ago learnt to avoid them.

There are excellent allergy cookbooks (some listed below) which give ideas for those who have many and varied sensitivities. The recipes included here are milk free, since that is our most common allergen; some are egg free and sugar free; all are free of artificial colours, flavours and preservatives. That does not mean that all are suitable for everyone (for instance, many milk allergic children may not eat cheese)—but at least it's a start. You can gradually reduce the variety of sweet and salted foods at your parties over time—children do come to enjoy natural foods when attractively presented.

Contact an allergy group for other ideas. If you know of none, write to Allergy Association Australia. (See last page.)

Some of the recipes included in this book are used with permission from *'Whole Foods For The Whole Family'*, La Leche League International, (1981), 9616 Minneapolis Ave., Franklin Park, Illinois 60131, USA.

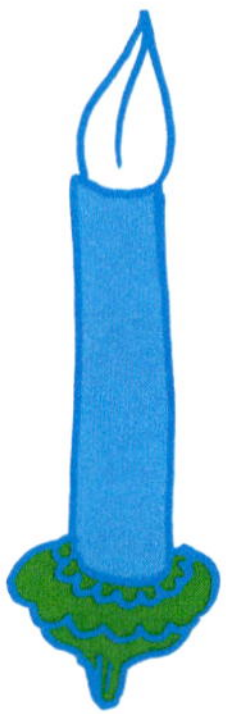

PARTY RECIPES FOR FOOD SENSITIVE CHILDREN

1. Michael's Birthday Cake
2. Alternative birthday cake
   (Milkless, sugarless, eggless, carrot cake)
3. Fruit sweets
4. Fantastic carob fudge
5. Honey crackles
6. Carob crackles
7. Picture salads
8. Yoghurt parfaits
9. Ice-cream
10. Drinks and icy-poles
11. Frozen bananas
12. Fruit salad
13. Barbecue

MICHAEL'S BIRTHDAY CAKE

1/2 cup margarine
3/4 cup honey
2 eggs
1 1/2 cups stewed or pureed apples
1 cup chopped apples
2 cups wholemeal S.R. flour
1 1/2 tsp cinnamon
1/4 tsp ground cloves
1/2 tsp nutmeg
1/2 tsp mixed spice
3/4 cup raisins or sultanas
3/4 cup walnuts or extra dried fruit

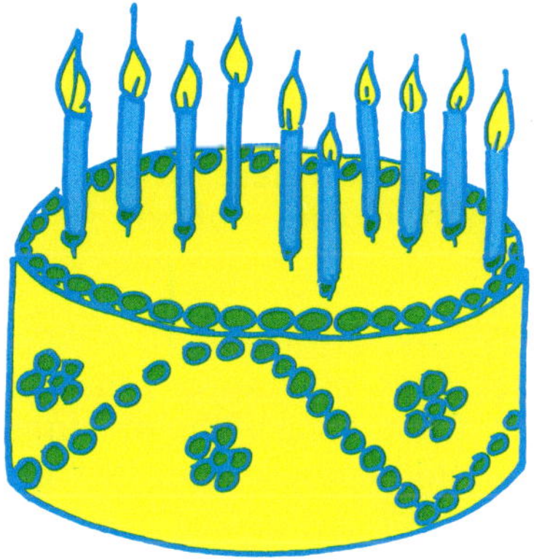

Michael's Birthday Cake

Decorate with:
sultanas, cinnamon, sesame seeds, nuts, raisins, sultanas, carob chips, candles in holders.
Natural colourings:
cochineal, blackcurrant juice, lemon juice, spinach juice, parsley juice.

Cream butter and honey together. Add eggs and stewed apples, and mix until smooth. Mix flour with other dry ingredients and add gradually to mixture. Beat briefly, then add the chunked apples. Stir in raisins or sultanas and nuts (if used). Pour into greased floured 9" (23cms) cake pan. Bake at 180° for 45-60 mins.

Adapted from 'Lisa's Wedding Cake', '*Whole Foods For the Whole Family*', LLLI.

HONEY FROSTING

1/3 cup honey
2-4 egg whites
dash of cream of tartar
1 tsp vanilla or almond essence

Combine all ingredients. Beat at high speed until fluffy. Use as frosting on 'Michael's Birthday Cake'.

EGGLESS, SUGARLESS, CARROT CAKE

1/2 cup grated carrots
1 1/4 cups dates—chopped
1 1/3 cups raisins
1/4 cup margarine (Nuttelex is milk free)
1 tsp each ground cinnamon, cloves, nutmeg
1 cup SR flour
1 cup SR wholemeal flour
1 1/2 cups chopped nuts or extra fruit

Place carrots, dates, water, fruit, margarine and spices in a pan. Bring slowly to boil and simmer for 5 minutes. Cool. Meanwhile stir together dry ingredients and add with nuts to first mixture. Stir until blended. Pour into greased and floured 9'' ring mould. Bake at 190° for 45-50 minutes.

Adapted from 'Eggless, Sugarless, Carrot Cake', *'Whole Foods for the Whole Family',* LLLI.

HONEY, CREAM CHEESE FILLING OR ICING

2 oz cream cheese
(cream cheese made from goat's milk is available for children allergic to cow's milk)
1 tablespoon Nuttelex margarine
3 tablespoons honey
1 tsp vanilla

Beat together and spread over cake.

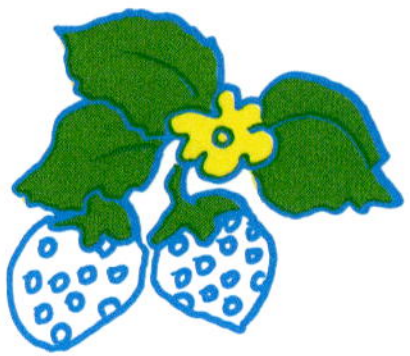

FRUIT SWEETS

Soak 1/4 cup raisins in 1/3 cup apple juice. Blend with 1/4 cup chopped dates and mix in 1 cup ground almonds and peanuts. Form into small balls.

FANTASTIC CAROB FUDGE

1/2-1 cup honey
1 cup peanut butter
1 cup carob powder
1 cup nuts, chopped, or seeds
1/2 tsp vanilla
Optional:
1 cup coconut
1/2 wheat germ

Put honey and peanut butter in a pan and stir over a low heat. Add carob powder, nuts, vanilla and coconut or wheat germ. Mix well. Spread mixture into a pan and refrigerate for one hour. When ready, cut into bite size pieces and enjoy.

Hint: When using carob powder melt or heat in oil or water. This makes it taste more like chocolate.

HONEY CRACKLES

2 tablespoons honey
3 tablespoons Nuttelex margarine
5-6 cups cornflakes or rice flakes
1/2 cup sultanas

Place margarine, honey and sugar in saucepan. Bring to the boil and cook for 1 minute. Remove from heat and stir in cornflakes and sultanas. Place in paper patty pans and bake in moderate oven for 8-10 minutes until slightly brown.
Makes about 16.

CAROB CRACKLES

Make as for chocolate crackles using carob instead of cocoa.

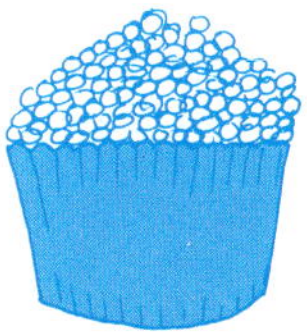

PICTURE SALADS

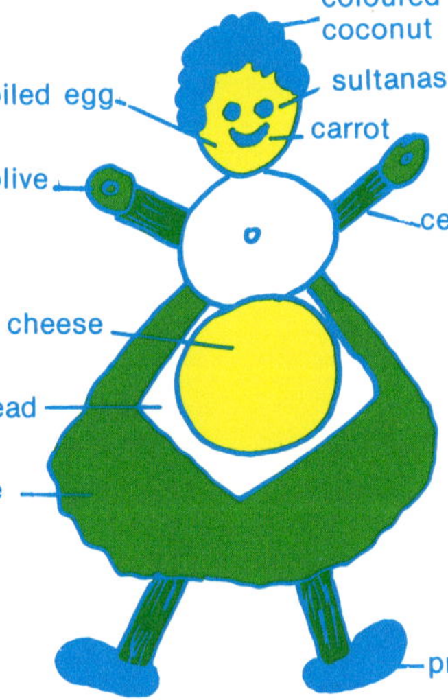

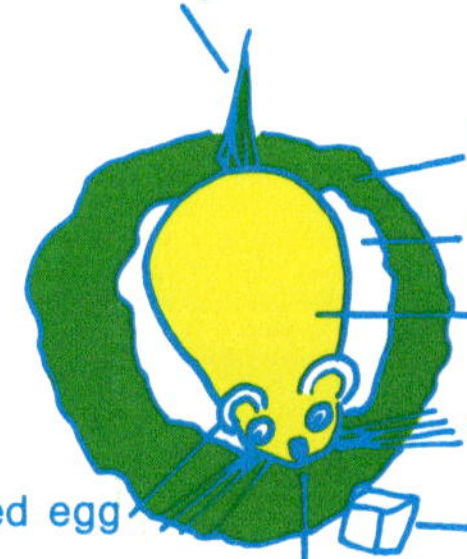

(Courtesy LLLI *'Whole Foods For The Whole Family'*)

YOGHURT PARFAITS

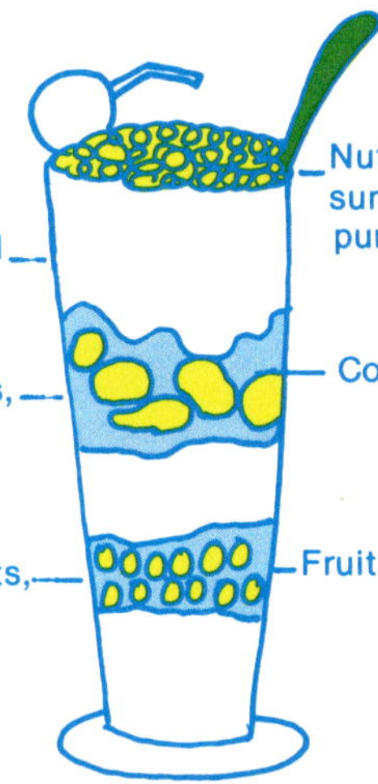

ICE CREAM

using no dairy products or sugar (no cooking required)

6 large, very ripe bananas
3 tablespoons maple syrup or
  2 tablespoons honey
2 tablespoons carob powder
1/3 cold-pressed oil (from health food shop)
4 tablespoons soya milk powder
1/3 cup water

Place all ingredients in blender and blend thoroughly. When liquified pour into refrigerator container, cover and place in freezer. It does not require a second beating.

Alternatives: The carob powder may be replaced by a handful of dates, or soaked seedless raisins. Serves 6-8.

DRINKS AND ICY-POLES

Our 'party' drinks include:

- Mountain Maid apple cider (preservative free)
- Apple, pear, or other juice mixed 50/50 with mineral water or carbonated water
- Doncaster fruit syrups heavily diluted (have preservatives, but are free of colours etc).

All of these make good icy poles—though there are now some commercial brands (too much sugar, but colour etc. free) which are occasionally tolerable. To be frozen, fruit juices etc. need to be a bit more concentrated than for drinking.

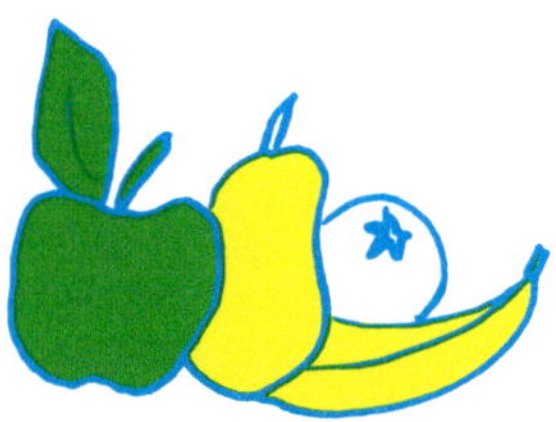

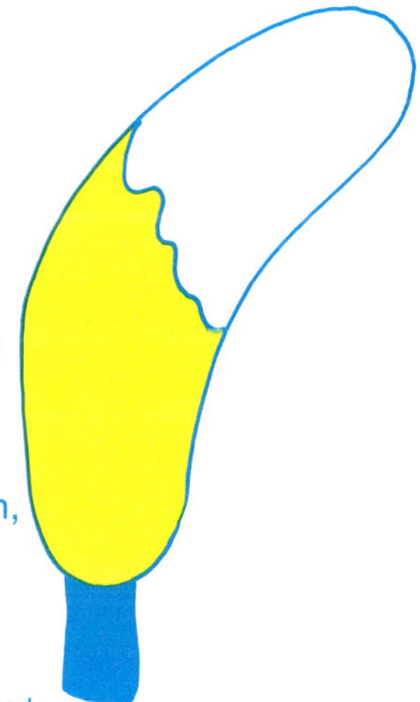

Frozen Bananas

Yoghurt—natural, coloured with cochineal and flavoured with crushed strawberries.

Other dips: peanut butter, wheat germ, crushed nuts, seeds, pureed fruits, coconut.

(Courtesy LLLI)

Further reading:

Food for Thought: a parent's guide to food intolerance. M. Minchin. (Alma Publications, 1982), $5 posted in Australia, (or $2 to low income families).
This contains an up to date resources list, bibliography, especially for Australian families. Its chief focus is the identification and management of food intolerances, with an emphasis on prevention—hence information about diet in pregnancy and while breastfeeding, and much more besides. Foreword by Prof. J. W. Gerrard, Dept. of Paediatric Allergy, University of Saskatchewan, Canada.
11,000 sold in 8 months without commercial distribution.

Tracking down hidden food allergy. W. Crook, M.D. (Professional Books, P.O. Box 3494, Jackson, Tennessee, U.S.A.) U.S. $7 posted.
The advantage of this book is its cartoon format, large print, and simple style. May help parents who would find *Food for Thought* too concentrated. However, it is not fully up to date, and is American.

Clinical Reactions to Food. (ed) M. H. Lessof (John Wiley & Sons, 1983) £24.95.
A very good review for professionals and parents used to medical language. Articles by specialists aware of controversies, but intelligent enough to take patients seriously.

Two essential addresses:

—for allergy information: Allergy Association Australia (AAA). Addresses of local groups, library facilities, etc.: P.O. Box 298, Ringwood, Vic., 3134.

—for breastfeeding information and support: Nursing Mothers' Association of Australia (NMAA), P.O. Box 231, Nunawading, Vic., 3131.

There are other relevant parent support groups; most are listed in *Food for Thought*. These are included as a starting point only.